# COMPLETE GUIDE TO COCHLEAR IMPLANT SURGERY

Comprehensive Manual To Advanced Techniques, Patient Care, And Optimized Outcomes For Hearing Restoration

## DR. BRUNO HORAN

# Disclaimer:

The information provided in this book, is intended for general informational purposes only and should not be considered as professional advice.

The author has made every effort to ensure the accuracy of the information presented. However, readers are advised to consult with a qualified healthcare professional before attempting any herbal remedies or making significant changes to their wellness routine. Individual health conditions vary, and what may be suitable for one person may not be appropriate for another.

It is important to note that the author is not in any endorsement deal, partnership, or affiliation with any organization, brand, or company mentioned in this book. Any references to specific products or services are based on the author's personal experience or general knowledge and do not imply an endorsement or promotion of those products or services

# Contents

# CONCERNING THIS BOOK

A priceless resource, "Cochlear Implant Surgery" carefully walks readers through the complex process of comprehending, undergoing, and adjusting to cochlear implants. The book starts by exploring the basic elements of hearing loss, providing a thorough synopsis of its different forms, underlying causes, and related risk factors. The book begins by explaining the significant impact that hearing loss can have on day-to-day activities. It then goes on to provide a thorough overview of cochlear implants, emphasizing both their advantages and inherent drawbacks. This section gives readers a strong basis for understanding the life-changing possibilities of cochlear implants and demystifies the complex nature of hearing loss.

Delving deeper into cochlear implants, the book provides a thorough breakdown of how these devices operate, clarifying the requirements for eligibility and dissecting the many parts of a cochlear implant system. It provides information about the anticipated results of the process, assisting prospective candidates in setting reasonable expectations for the capabilities of cochlear implants. For individuals who are thinking about the process, this part is essential because it sets expectations and provides education, which helps people make well-informed decisions.

Equal attention to detail is devoted to the pre-operative phase, bringing readers through the early consultations and assessments required before the procedure. It highlights how crucial it is to evaluate one's medical history, get preoperative exams and scans, and take insurance coverage and cost into account. To guarantee that potential patients are completely ready for the life-altering event ahead, the book also discusses the sometimes disregarded topic of mental and emotional preparedness.

A step-by-step description of the surgical procedure is provided, including everything from the options for anesthetic and safety precautions to the surgical methods and tools utilized. Along with postoperative care recommendations, the discussion of potential risks and problems offers a realistic and comforting summary of what to expect both during and after the surgery. For patients and their families, this portion is priceless since it provides clarity and comfort.

During the crucial stages of recovery and rehabilitation associated with a cochlear implant, the book provides comprehensive advice on post-surgery care, pain management, and implant activation. Exercises and rehabilitation plans are described to help the patient get used to their new hearing experience. Follow-up visits and continuous monitoring guarantee that the patient's progress is maintained. The dedication needed for a successful implant adaption is emphasized in this section.

Constant adaptation is required when living with a cochlear implant; this book offers helpful guidance on communication tactics, setting up the environment, and maintaining the device.

Included are links for support networks and troubleshooting assistance, highlighting the significance of adopting a comprehensive approach to living with an implant. This section offers implant users a wealth of useful guidance and assistance.

The book addresses typical concerns by addressing issues with long-term effectiveness, psychological changes, compatibility with other medical devices, and influence on speech and language development.

It also discusses social acceptability and stigma, giving readers coping skills and approaches to deal with these problems. This section is especially helpful in clearing up misconceptions and offering comfort.

Common inquiries concerning eligibility, age restrictions, the length of operation, and the use of hearing aids are addressed in a FAQ section. For anyone looking for precise solutions to questions regarding cochlear implants, it offers rapid and easily accessible information. This useful section makes the book a more valuable resource.

The book closes with a look ahead at ongoing treatment and potential advancements in the cochlear implant industry.

It covers regular upkeep, repairing and updating gadget parts, as well as new developments in research and upcoming technologies. The emphasis on advocacy and community involvement also encourages readers to get involved in larger campaigns to promote and advance the accessibility and technology of cochlear implants.

# CHAPTER ONE

## COMPASSION FOR HEARING LOSS

### Types Of Hearing Loss

Three primary types of hearing loss are generally recognized: mixed, sensorineural, and conductive. When there is a problem with the middle or outer ear that stops sound from being conducted to the inner ear, it is known as conductive hearing loss.

Ear infections, middle ear fluid, ear wax accumulation, and structural abnormalities of the ear are common reasons.

Damage to the cochlea, the inner ear, or the auditory nerve pathways leading to the brain can result in sensorineural hearing loss.

These can be brought on by aging, exposure to loud noises, head trauma, or certain medications. They are typically permanent.

A combination of sensorineural and conductive hearing loss, known as mixed hearing loss, denotes issues with the auditory nerve or inner ear as well as the middle or outer ear.

## Reasons And Danger Elements

Numerous events and risk factors can lead to hearing loss. In particular, when it comes to congenital hearing loss that is evident from birth, genetic factors are important.

Presbycusis, or aging, is a natural process that frequently begins at age 60. Another important component is noise exposure, especially from extended exposure to loud noises from industrial, events, or headphones.

Measles, mumps, and meningitis are among the infections that can cause hearing loss. Certain antibiotics and chemotherapy treatments are examples of ototoxic medications that can harm the inner ear. Chronic ear infections, head trauma, and medical disorders including hypertension and diabetes can all cause hearing loss.

## Effects On Day-To-Day Living

The quality of life of an individual can be significantly impacted by hearing loss. When communication is difficult, social isolation and mental suffering are common outcomes.

Particularly in noisy settings, people with hearing loss may find it difficult to follow discussions, which can cause irritation and misunderstandings.

 This may have an impact on social interactions, educational success, and job performance. Untreated hearing loss increases the likelihood of dementia and cognitive decline in affected persons.

When it gets harder to hear traffic sounds, warning signals, or sirens, there is a greater chance of accidents, which raises safety concerns.

# Overview Of Cochlear Implants

Cochlear implants are advanced medical devices that give people with severe to profound sensorineural hearing loss—who do not get enough benefit from traditional hearing aids—a perception of sound.

Cochlear implants stimulate the auditory nerve directly, avoiding damaged parts of the ear, in contrast to hearing aids that amplify sounds.

 The gadget is composed of two parts: an exterior part that is positioned behind the ear and a second part that is surgically inserted beneath the skin.

The interior portion has an electrode array that is implanted into the cochlea and a receiver, while the external portion consists of a microphone, speech processor, and transmitter.

# Advantages And Drawbacks

Cochlear implants have many advantages. They can greatly enhance voice comprehension and environmental sound perception, which will increase social interactions and communication.

Numerous beneficiaries report having a higher quality of life and feeling more confident going about their everyday lives. When placed in children at an early age, cochlear implants can help with speech and language development, especially for those with substantial hearing loss.

There are restrictions, though. The results of cochlear implants can vary based on factors such as the age of implantation, length of deafness, and pre-implant hearing ability. Cochlear implants do not restore normal hearing.

Some people could still struggle to enjoy music and background noise. The procedure and equipment are expensive, and while insurance may partially reimburse the costs, there may be substantial out-of-pocket expenditures.

To guarantee proper function, the implant also needs to be maintained regularly and monitored for the rest of one's life.

Being aware of these factors enables people to manage their hearing loss and weigh the pros and downsides of cochlear implants.

# CHAPTER TWO

## INVESTIGATING CHLORINE IMPLANTS

### Functions Of Cochlear Implants

Cochlear implants are advanced medical devices that let people with severe to profound hearing loss perceive sound.

Cochlear implants stimulate the auditory nerve directly, avoiding damaged parts of the ear, in contrast to hearing aids that amplify sound. This is accomplished by a series of steps:

Sound Collection: The device's external microphone, which is often worn behind the ear, records sound.

Sound processing: A speech processor receives the recorded sound and uses digital technology to evaluate and convert it into coded signals.

Transmission to Implant: An electrode array that is surgically put into the cochlea is connected to the internal implant, which receives these signals via a coil.

Electrical Stimulation: Electrical impulses are used by the electrode array to activate the cochlea's auditory nerve fibers.

Interpretation of Signals: These signals are then sent by the auditory nerve to the brain, where they are deciphered as familiar sounds.

People who are deaf or very hard of hearing may now experience sound thanks to this complex technology, which improves their ability to communicate and interact with their surroundings.

# The Cochlear Implant System's Components

The external and internal components of a cochlear implant device function in unison to enhance hearing.

Outside Elements:

Microphone: Record audio from surrounding sources.

Speech processor: Generates a digital signal from sound. It may be adjusted to meet the demands of the user and is commonly worn on the body or behind the ear.

Transmitter Coil: Uses radio waves to transmit a digital signal via the skin to an inside receiver.

Inside Parts:

Under the skin, a device known as a receiver stimulator takes signals from an external transmitter and transforms them into electrical impulses.

An array of small  electrodes that are surgically placed inside the cochlea. The sense of sound is produced by these electrodes stimulating the fibers of the auditory nerve.

Each part is essential to ensure that sound is converted and transmitted smoothly, enabling users to efficiently take in and interpret auditory information.

Qualifications

Cochlear implants are not appropriate for all hearing-impaired people. To guarantee that the user will get something from the device, certain requirements must be fulfilled:

Degree of Hearing Loss: Candidates usually have sensorineural (damage to the inner ear or auditory nerve) hearing loss in both ears, ranging from severe to profound.

Limited Benefit from Hearing Aids:

When candidates wear traditional hearing aids, they typically experience very slight improvements, which suggests that the amplification is insufficient.

General Health: To have surgery, a candidate must be in good health and free from any illnesses that could make the process more difficult.

Cochlear Structure: For the implant to be successful, there must be a functional auditory nerve and sufficient cochlear structure.

Age considerations: Early implantation in children can greatly improve speech and language development, although adults and children as young as 12 months old can be candidates.

Motivation and Support: To benefit from the rehabilitation procedure, which includes post-surgery therapy and adjustments, candidates and their families must be devoted and driven.

An otologist, audiologist, and other medical specialists evaluate candidates in-depth to ascertain the possible advantages of the implant for each candidate.

Anticipated Results

Depending on several variables, including the recipient's age at implantation, the severity of their hearing loss, and the state of their auditory nerve, cochlear implant outcomes can differ greatly amongst recipients. In general, recipients should anticipate:

Enhanced Sound Awareness: The majority of users report a noticeable increase in their capacity to distinguish between a variety of sounds, such as speech and background noise.

Better Speech Understanding: Over time, many receivers report that they can understand speech in both quiet and noisy settings.

Better Communication: People who have better hearing frequently have better communication skills, which facilitate smoother and more fruitful exchanges.

Quality of Life: Due to their increased ability to participate fully in social, educational, and professional activities, many users report an overall improvement in their quality of life.

Even though results can be extremely favorable, they depend on the user's dedication to post-implantation rehabilitation and consistent device use.

## Reasonable Anticipations

Anyone thinking about getting a cochlear implant needs to be sure they have reasonable expectations. It's critical to realize that:

The First Sounds Might Not Be Familiar: The brain requires some time to get used to the new sense of hearing.

Though they could seem robotic or hazy at first, these sounds usually get better with time and practice.

Continued Therapy Is Critical: Post-implantation speech and hearing therapy is necessary to maximize results. Through this therapy, users' speech comprehension improves and they learn how to understand the new sounds.

Frequent Device Maintenance: To guarantee optimum performance, the cochlear implant's exterior components require periodic upgrades and routine maintenance.

Differential Outcomes: Cochlear implant success can differ. While some users may reach hearing levels close to normal, others might still need to rely on lipreading or other forms of communication.

 Results can vary depending on factors like the age at implantation and the length of deafness.

Continuous Adaptation: To preserve the optimal hearing experience, speech processor settings will need to be changed as technology and the user's auditory ability advance.

Comprehending these facets facilitates the establishment of a practical structure for prospective recipients and their relatives, guaranteeing that they are equipped for the forthcoming cochlear implant expedition.

# CHAPTER THREE

## GETTING READY FOR SURGERY

### First Consultations And Assessments

Complete consultations and examinations are the first steps on the path to cochlear implant surgery. The medical team will evaluate if the implant is appropriate for the patient during these initial consultations. During these consultations, the patient's hearing history, present auditory ability, and any prior interventions or treatments are usually thoroughly discussed. To assess the degree of hearing loss and the functionality of any residual natural hearing, the audiologist will perform a battery of hearing tests. This stage is essential because it creates a baseline from which the efficacy of the cochlear implant can be evaluated after surgery.

In addition, the structural components of the ear will be examined by an ENT specialist. This could entail looking inside the eardrum and canal under a microscope to make sure there are no infections or obstructions that could make surgery more difficult. To ensure the best potential outcome, these examinations are thorough and customized to give a clear picture of the patient's candidacy for the implant.

## Evaluation Of Medical History

An extensive evaluation of one's medical history is essential to getting ready for cochlear implant surgery. During this procedure, comprehensive data regarding the patient's general health, past surgeries, prescriptions, allergies, and any ongoing medical issues must be gathered. Finding any possible hazards or contraindications that can affect the procedure or the healing process is the aim of this assessment.

Questions regarding blood clotting disorders, diabetes, heart ailments, and other systemic health issues will be posed to the patients. The surgical team can better predict and manage any issues during and after the procedure with the use of this information. Knowing the patient's medical background enables the creation of a personalized surgical plan that addresses their unique medical requirements, guaranteeing a safer and more successful procedure.

## Preoperative Examinations And Mris

The process of getting ready for cochlear implant surgery must include preoperative exams and scans. These examinations offer comprehensive information about the structure of the ear and the patient's general state of health. Common tests that yield high-resolution images of the inner ear structures are magnetic resonance imaging (MRI) and computed tomography (CT) scans. The surgical team can more precisely plan the implant's location with the aid of these scans.

Blood tests are also performed to look for any underlying medical issues, such as anemia or infections, that could interfere with the procedure. To verify the degree of hearing loss and create a final baseline for comparisons after surgery, audiometric testing is repeated. Before the procedure, these thorough examinations guarantee that every facet of the patient's health and ear anatomy is recognized.

## Insurance And Financial Aspects

A vital part of being ready is navigating the financial implications of cochlear implant surgery. Patients must be aware of all the expenses involved in the procedure, including those for the implant device, the hospital, anesthesia, and follow-up visits. It's critical to go over these prices with the healthcare practitioner and obtain an accurate assessment of the overall costs.

The provider and the patient's particular plan will determine how much coverage is provided by insurance. To find out what parts of the cochlear implant procedure are covered, patients should get in touch with their insurance provider. Certain plans might pay the full amount, while others would only pay a fraction of it. It's also worthwhile to look into any grants or financial aid programs that might be accessible to people who meet the requirements. Patients can focus on their surgical preparation and recuperation by reducing stress and being aware of these financial factors upfront.

## Emotional And Mental Preparedness

One of the most important aspects of getting ready for cochlear implant surgery is mental and emotional preparation. The choice to have such surgery done might elicit a variety of feelings, from anticipation and hope to fear and anxiety. Patients must be emotionally and psychologically ready for both the surgery and the period of recovery that follows.

It is recommended that patients talk about their feelings and concerns with mental health specialists as well as their family and friends. Counseling programs can offer a secure setting for discussing any worries you may have about the operation and the adjustments it will entail. It might be helpful to join support groups for persons who have had cochlear implant surgery since they offer a network of people who have been there before and can offer both emotional and practical support.

Patients' ability to recuperate and acclimate to the cochlear implant can be greatly impacted by their mental and emotional readiness, which enables them to face the procedure with resilience and a positive outlook.

# CHAPTER FOUR

## THE SURGICAL METHOD

### A Comprehensive Synopsis Of The Procedure

A careful procedure called cochlear implant surgery is used to help people with severe to profound hearing loss regain their hearing. To expose the mastoid bone, the surgeon makes a little incision behind the ear at the start of the treatment. To gain access to the middle ear, the surgeon makes a tiny incision in the bone using a high-precision drill. The electrode array must next be carefully inserted into the cochlea, the spiral-shaped inner ear structure that sends sound information to the brain. The receiver-stimulator device is fastened beneath the skin and muscles above the ear by the surgeon once the electrode array is positioned. The cochlea's electrodes will receive signals from this device, which will then relay them to the external processor. Following imaging procedures to confirm proper placement, the surgeon stitches the incision closed and wraps it with a sterile bandage.

## Options For Anesthesia And Safety Precautions

Anesthesia is essential for maintaining the patient's comfort and safety during cochlear implant surgery. Usually, general anesthesia is given, which keeps the patient unconscious and pain-free for the duration of the operation. To reduce the hazards associated with general anesthesia, local anesthetic combined with sedation may be used in certain instances, particularly for adult patients.

Throughout the procedure, an anesthesiologist continuously checks vital signs like blood pressure, oxygen saturation, and heart rate. This monitoring aids in quickly resolving any potential problems. Preoperative evaluations are carried out to ascertain the most suitable anesthesia strategy for every patient, guaranteeing individualized and secure care.

These evaluations include a comprehensive medical history and any required lab testing.

## Instruments And Procedures For Surgery

Sophisticated surgical methods and specialized equipment are critical to the success of cochlear implant surgery. Surgical loupes and high-definition microscopes help surgeons see better throughout the procedure's minute details.

The incision is made in the mastoid bone using precision drills, and the electrode array is gently inserted into the cochlea with the help of small, flexible devices.

To verify that the electrodes are positioned correctly inside the cochlea and to test the implant's performance, electrophysiological monitoring techniques are used.

Real-time feedback is made possible by this technology, which aids in maximizing the implant's alignment and placement for optimum auditory results. Before the procedure is finished, imaging techniques such as intraoperative CT scans or X-rays may also be utilized to verify the implant's location.

## Possible Dangers And Issues

As with any surgical treatment, cochlear implant surgery has some risks and potential problems even though it is generally safe and successful. Bleeding, anesthesia-related responses, and surgical site infection are common hazards.

Patients may occasionally have transient problems with balance or dizziness as a result of the inner ear components' proximity. face nerve damage is a less common consequence that can lead to either acute or chronic face muscle paralysis.

Furthermore, there is a remote chance that the implant device will malfunction and require additional surgery. Patients and their caregivers should be aware of these risks in advance of the procedure and should also be aware of the warning signs of potential problems, which include fever, edema, or chronic discomfort that would need to be treated right away.

## Instructions For Postoperative Care

After cochlear implant surgery, proper postoperative care is essential to a speedy recovery and the best possible results. Patients are kept under close observation in the recovery room until they fully recover from the treatment and their vital signs stabilize. Instructions on how to care for the region around the incision should be given, and the surgical site needs to be kept dry and clean. Prescription drugs may be used in pain management to reduce discomfort.

To allow for adequate healing, patients are usually recommended to refrain from heavy lifting and vigorous activity for a few weeks. Appointments for follow-up are planned to track the healing process and turn on the cochlear implant. Patients receive fittings and programming for the external processor during these appointments, and they start working with a team of speech therapists and audiologists for auditory rehabilitation.

To achieve optimal hearing outcomes, it is imperative to stick to the specified rehabilitation plan and receive consistent follow-up care.

# CHAPTER FIVE

## REPAY AND RESUMMATION

### Immediate Care Following Surgery:

To guarantee a speedy recovery following cochlear implant surgery, it's imperative to adhere to the recommended post-operative care instructions.

You're probably going to feel a little sore and swollen in the area where the procedure was performed. Your medical team will provide you with advice on how to properly treat these symptoms.

Keeping the surgical site dry and clean is a major part of immediate post-surgery care. You will receive detailed instructions from your healthcare practitioner on how to take care of the incision site, including when and how to change dressings, if needed. To stop infection and encourage recovery, it's critical to adhere to these directions precisely.

In addition, your medical staff might recommend painkillers to help you cope with any post-operative discomfort. It's critical to take these drugs as prescribed and to notify your healthcare provider right away if you experience any severe or ongoing pain. For your body to recuperate effectively during this period, rest is also essential.

## Handling Soreness And Pain:

After cochlear implant surgery, pain and discomfort are common, but there are a few tactics you can use to effectively manage these symptoms.

To help with discomfort throughout the healing process, your healthcare practitioner could provide painkillers.

You must take these drugs exactly as prescribed and let your healthcare provider know if you have any unfavorable side effects.

Ice packs applied to the surgery site can aid with pain relief and edema reduction in addition to medication. Make sure you adhere to the advice from your healthcare professional regarding how often and how long to use ice packs.

Another essential element of controlling pain and discomfort following cochlear implant surgery is rest. A seamless recovery depends on avoiding demanding activities and giving your body time to recover. Pay attention to your body's signals and allow yourself the time and room you require for a complete recovery.

## Cochlear Implant Activation:

After the initial healing phase, which usually lasts two to four weeks following surgery, you will go through the cochlear implant activation procedure.

This entails setting up the gadget to produce sound perception and stimulate the auditory nerve.

Your audiologist will modify the cochlear implant's settings at the activation visit to your unique hearing requirements and preferences. Your audiologist will adjust the device to maximize your hearing experience, which could take several hours.

It may take some time to become used to the new sounds that the cochlear implant provides, so it's important to approach the activation procedure patiently and with an open mind. Throughout this process, your audiologist will offer advice and assistance to help you get used to your newfound hearing.

## Exercises And Programs For Rehabilitation:

You will take part in rehabilitation programs and exercises once your cochlear implant is activated to help you reach your full hearing potential. Speech therapy, listening practice sessions, and auditory training exercises are some of the programs that may be included.

The goal of the auditory training exercises is to teach you how to appropriately interpret the sounds that your cochlear implant produces.

In these tasks, listening to numerous sounds and differentiating between speech sounds, tones, and pitches may be required.

Those who have had cochlear implant surgery may also benefit from speech therapy, especially if they have had hearing loss since a young age. The main goals of speech therapy sessions are to enhance vocabulary, understanding, and articulation, among other speech and language abilities.

People with cochlear implants can practice applying their newfound sense of hearing in natural environments by participating in listening practice sessions. To enhance listening comprehension and communication skills, these sessions may entail watching movies, taking part in group discussions, or listening to conversations.

Subsequent Meetings and Observation:

Following cochlear implant surgery and activation, you will have routine follow-up appointments with your healthcare team so that your device can be adjusted as needed and to monitor your progress. These visits usually take place regularly in the first year after surgery and may decrease in frequency as you get used to using your cochlear implant.

Your audiologist will perform a battery of tests during these follow-up visits to evaluate your hearing capacity and make sure your cochlear implant is operating as intended.

In addition, they might modify the device's programming in response to your comments and any modifications to your hearing requirements.

Attending all of your planned follow-up appointments is crucial. You should also be honest with your healthcare staff about any worries you may have about your cochlear implant.

Working together with your audiologist and other medical professionals, you can make sure you get the help and support you require to get the most out of your cochlear implant.

# CHAPTER SIX

## COPING WITH IMPLANT COCHLEAR

### Adjusting To Cochlear Implant Hearing:

Comprehending the Process of Adjustment:

Living with a cochlear implant can involve a journey of successes and challenges. It's normal to feel a range of emotions right after surgery, from excitement to anxiety. It takes time for the brain to adjust to processing sounds in a new way, particularly if you have been deaf or hard of hearing for a long time. Recall that throughout this time, patience is essential.

Gradual Advancement:

Getting used to a cochlear implant takes time. Voices may sound robotic at first, and noises may seem off or distorted. Your brain will, however, become more adept at deciphering these signals with time and experience. To prevent overtaxing your hearing system, you must heed the advice of your audiologist or hearing specialist regarding the steady rise in sound levels.

Rehabilitation of Communication:

It is essential to participate in communication rehabilitation programs if you want to get the most out of your cochlear implant. Speech therapy, auditory training, and listening exercises are frequently included in these programs to improve your ability to perceive and understand sounds. Your capacity to speak in a variety of contexts can be greatly improved with regularity and commitment to these programs.

## Techniques And Advice For Communication:

### Making Use of Visual Cues

When communicating, it can be quite helpful to use visual cues to help you understand speech, particularly in noisy settings or when you are speaking with someone whose accent is new to you. You can use gestures, lipreading, and facial expressions to provide important context to the auditory information your cochlear implant provides.

Speaking Up for Yourself:

Never be afraid to speak up in different situations for what you need in terms of communication. Sharing information with others about your cochlear implant and how they can support you in communicating better helps increase empathy and understanding. This could be asking speakers to face you directly or asking for a quieter setting when having conversations.

Engage in Active Listening:

Focusing on the speaker and attempting to comprehend what they are saying are both components of active listening. To increase your comprehension during conversations, try not to multitask or be distracted. Effective communication can also be improved by clarifying what you've heard and asking questions when necessary.

## Environmental Modifications:

Enhancing Your surroundings:

You can improve your overall cochlear implant listening experience by making changes to your surroundings. Clearer communication can be achieved by situating yourself closer to the speaker, employing assistive listening equipment like FM systems or captioning services, and minimizing background noise by using sound-absorbing materials.

Developing Areas That Encourage Communication:

Communication-focused design can improve the accessibility of everyday interactions in your home or place of business. To improve speech perception, build visual alert systems for doorbells and alarms, use captioned televisions or video calling platforms, and arrange furniture to minimize echo and reverberation.

Teaching Others:

Providing information to friends, family, coworkers, and educators about the particular environmental elements that affect hearing can help create a welcoming and supportive environment. Urge them to make little but effective changes, such as turning to face you when speaking, speaking clearly and slowly, and if at all possible, reducing background noise.

## Maintenance And Troubleshooting Of Devices:

Normal Upkeep and Care:

For your cochlear implant device to function at its best and last a long time, regular care and maintenance are required. This entails maintaining the integrity of the implant site by following recommended hygiene procedures and wiping down external components like the processor and microphone with a gentle cloth or specialized wipes.

Keeping an eye on the battery life:

It's essential to keep an eye on your cochlear implant processor's battery life to prevent unplanned hearing loss. To avoid downtime, become familiar with the battery indicators and change the batteries as needed. Having extra batteries on hand can give peace of mind, particularly while traveling or attending long events.

Troubleshooting Typical Problems:

You might occasionally experience problems with your cochlear implant system, even with your best efforts. Learn how to troubleshoot using the methods your audiologist or manufacturer suggests, such as restarting the processor, looking for damage or blockages in the components, and making sure the accessories are connected properly.

Looking for Assistance:

While living with a cochlear implant can be empowering, difficulties are common while adjusting to it. Never be afraid to ask for help from advocacy groups, support groups, internet forums, and other cochlear implant recipients. Guidance and encouragement can be gained from others' experiences and shared.

Getting to Know Educational Resources:

Use reliable resources to educate yourself about cochlear implants and hearing loss, including medical practitioners, scholarly publications, and instructional websites. Gaining knowledge about the technology underlying cochlear implants, the procedure, and continuing therapy will help you become an advocate for yourself and make well-informed decisions.

Making Use of Rehabilitation Services:

Utilize the rehabilitation services that your hearing healthcare team or audiologist has to offer. These could be customized instructional seminars, group workshops, and individual therapy sessions based on your requirements and objectives. Increasing the number of experts in your field who are familiar with cochlear implants will help you on your path to improved hearing.

# CHAPTER SEVEN

## TAKING CARE OF COMMON ISSUES

### Effects On Language And Speech Development

Speech and language development are greatly improved with cochlear implants, especially in the case of early implant placement.

These gadgets stimulate the auditory nerve directly, avoiding damaged ear tissue and enabling the brain to receive sound impulses.

Because early implantation makes use of the brain's flexibility, it can improve speech and language acquisition.

To get the most out of the implant, children typically go through extensive speech therapy after surgery. The child's therapists work with them to enhance their articulation, listening comprehension, and listening abilities. Improved speech perception may also be experienced by adults obtaining implants, though results may differ depending on the severity and length of hearing loss previous to surgery.

## Adaptability To Different Medical Devices

Although cochlear implants are made to work with a variety of medical equipment, it's still vital to disclose the device to medical professionals before any treatments.

For example, MRI devices may cause interference with the implant; however, under certain circumstances, newer versions of cochlear implants are frequently MRI-compatible.

Additionally, patients should exercise caution when using certain dental tools, electrotherapy devices, and hearing aids.

Comprehensive instructions on how to use various medical equipment securely in conjunction with a cochlear implant can be obtained by consulting audiologists and the implant manufacturer.

## Long-Term Durability And Effectiveness

Cochlear implants are designed to last a lifetime and offer long-term hearing aids. The surgically inserted inside component is meant to last a lifetime. However, as technology develops, the external processor might need to be upgraded or replaced regularly.

It is essential to schedule routine follow-up visits to assess the implant's functionality and make any required modifications.

These check-ins guarantee that the device is operating at peak efficiency and that any new features or software updates can be applied to improve the user experience.

Many beneficiaries note that these developments have led to ongoing improvements in their hearing over time.

# Psychological Modifications And Coping Strategies

There are major psychological adjustments involved in becoming used to a cochlear implant. Users may initially experience a sense of overwhelm due to the novel auditory experiences and the learning curve involved in deciphering these sounds. It is crucial to have professional, familial, and friend support throughout this time.

Support groups and counseling can be quite helpful in assisting people in managing the emotional aspects of hearing loss and the switch to implant use.

These tools offer a forum for exchanging experiences, stress-reduction techniques, and creating a caring community.

## Acceptance And Social Stigma

For many recipients, the social stigma associated with cochlear implants can be a source of concern. Feelings of loneliness or self-consciousness can result from misconceptions about the device or hearing loss. To mitigate these concerns, education and awareness are essential.

Recipients must have candid conversations about their experiences since doing so helps demystify the technology and foster acceptance. Workplaces, social settings, and schools should all be inclusive spaces that provide accommodations and promote understanding. As more people learn about the advantages of cochlear implants, social acceptance of them grows with time.

# CHAPTER EIGHT

## COMMON QUESTIONS ANSWERED (FAQS)

### Who Is Eligible For A Cochlear Implant?

Cochlear implants are not appropriate for every person. Those with severe to profound sensorineural hearing loss in both ears who find little to no gain from conventional hearing aids are usually considered candidates. To evaluate if a patient is a good candidate for an implant, a comprehensive medical examination, audiological evaluations, and imaging examinations are conducted. Other factors taken into account are the length of the hearing loss, the cochlea's structure, and general health.

If a person's hearing aids don't allow them enough clarity or comprehension of speech, they may still be a candidate for a cochlear implant. Both adults and pediatric patients may be candidates, however for the implant to be helpful, certain requirements must be satisfied. To ascertain eligibility, a consultation with a specialist otolaryngologist and audiologist is required.

## What Is The Minimum Age To Receive A Cochlear Implant?

Age restrictions do not apply to cochlear implantation. If they are healthy and fit, older adults—including those in their 70s, 80s, and even 90s—can get cochlear implants. The person's general health and capacity to withstand anesthesia and surgery safely are the main concerns. With the successful placement of cochlear implants, many older persons have seen notable gains in their quality of life.

Cochlear implants can be placed in children as early as 12 months of age, while under some conditions, babies younger than a year old may also be candidates for them. Since early implantation gives children access to auditory input throughout the critical stages of speech and language acquisition, it can be extremely beneficial for language development. To make sure they will benefit from the implant, pediatric applicants go through a thorough screening that includes tests conducted by speech therapists, audiologists, and other medical specialists.

## What Is The Duration Of The Surgery?

Generally speaking, cochlear implant surgery takes two to four hours, depending on the surgeon's competence and the complexity of the case. Under general anesthesia, the treatment is carried out, and most patients can return home the same day, while some might need to stay overnight for observation.

During the procedure, a tiny incision is made behind the ear, the cochlea is punctured, and the electrode array is inserted. After that, the internal receiver is positioned beneath the skin. The surgical site must heal during the recovery phase following the procedure before the external components are attached and turned on, which typically happens two to four weeks after the procedure.

Can I continue to wear my hearing aids?

People who have had a cochlear implant can continue to wear hearing aids, particularly if they still retain hearing in their non-implanted ears. Combining the advantages of both technologies might result in a more realistic and rich sound experience, which is called bimodal hearing. The opposite ear can benefit from a hearing aid to increase general sound perception, find noises more easily, and comprehend speech in noisy surroundings.

Some patients may wear hearing aids in both ears before surgery, and after obtaining a cochlear implant, they may continue to wear them in the non-implanted ear. An audiologist evaluates and optimizes this dual use to guarantee the patient has the greatest potential hearing outcome.

Can someone with a cochlear implant shower or swim?

Yes, but there's a need for prudence. Because the internal parts of a cochlear implant are waterproof, you can shower and swim without any problems. But the external parts, like the microphone and CPU, aren't water resistant, so you have to take them out before doing anything that involves water.

There are specialized attachments and waterproof covers that can shield the external components to allow swimming and other water-based sports. Patients who want to prolong the life and functionality of their cochlear implants should always adhere to the manufacturer's instructions and seek guidance from their audiologist regarding the optimal ways to use these devices.

# CHAPTER NINE

## AFTER SURGERY: ONGOING CARE AND FUTURE ADVANCES

### Regular Upkeep And Post-Impact Care

Following cochlear implant surgery, follow-up checkups, and continued care are essential to ensuring patient satisfaction and the best possible device performance. To track the healing process, modify the external speech processor, and fine-tune the implant's settings, patients will initially need to make regular sessions. These appointments usually take place in the initial weeks following surgery and then progressively decrease in frequency as the patient becomes used to the device.

Cleaning the external parts, including the processor and microphone, is part of routine maintenance that helps to ensure good sound transmission and prevent damage. Patients receive instructions on how to handle these parts with caution and carry out simple troubleshooting, like making sure all the connections are made correctly and checking the battery levels. During these follow-up appointments, audiologists are crucial because they administer hearing tests to gauge progress and modify the implant's settings as needed. Frequent examinations of hearing are necessary to monitor the patient's development and swiftly address any issues.

## Modernizing And Replacing Electronic Parts

Cochlear implants keep up with technological advancements. Living with a cochlear implant often entails updating and replacing device components. New processors and accessories that provide better battery life, higher sound quality, and more user comfort are constantly being developed by manufacturers. These improvements can have a big impact on patients, yet updating only requires swapping out the external processor.

Although the internal implant itself is meant to survive for many years, due to developments in technology or device failure, it might eventually need to be replaced. Surgery might be necessary in some situations to replace the internal parts, however this is less frequent. It is recommended that patients be aware of advancements in cochlear implant technology and consult with their audiologists about possible updates to guarantee they are utilizing the most advanced and efficient equipment available.

## New Developments In Research And Emerging Technologies

The field of cochlear implants is developing quickly as engineers and researchers are always looking for new ways to improve users' auditory experiences. The application of artificial intelligence (AI) to sound processors is one fascinating field of research and development. AI can assist in the device's learning and adaptation to various listening contexts, resulting in improved sound quality and more efficient background noise reduction.

The creation of fully implanted cochlear implants, which do away with the requirement for an external processor entirely, is another encouraging development.

The goal of these gadgets is to provide users with better convenience and a more natural hearing experience. Furthermore, to improve sound quality and lower surgical risks, research is being done on electrode design and placement techniques.

Potential remedies for hearing loss are also being investigated, including gene therapy and stem cell research. Although these technologies are currently in the experimental phase, they have the potential to help people with specific forms of hearing loss regain their natural hearing, which could eventually lessen or eliminate the need for cochlear implants.

Being a cochlear implant user includes more than simply navigating the medical system; it also entails integrating into a strong, powerful community. The lives of people who utilize cochlear implants are significantly impacted by advocacy and community involvement. A plethora of organizations and support groups provide information, instruction, and a forum for people to share their stories and promote improved healthcare for hearing impairments.

To connect with other people who have experienced similar things, patients are encouraged to participate in these communities—whether in person or online. Engaging in advocacy endeavors may involve spreading knowledge about hearing impairment, advocating for prompt intervention, and endorsing laws that guarantee accessibility to hearing aids and technologies. Cochlear implant users can lessen the stigma attached to hearing loss and promote an inclusive society by sharing their experiences and obstacles.

## Having A Cochlear Implant And Leading A Happy Life

People with severe to profound hearing loss can live much better lives with a cochlear implant. Patients who can sense sounds may benefit from improved communication, a more fulfilling social life, and more chances for employment and education. Learning new listening techniques and, for some, honing spoken language skills are important parts of adjusting to life with a cochlear implant.

Following implantation, rehabilitation therapies including speech therapy and auditory training are frequently included. Through these programs, patients can enhance their communication abilities and learn to comprehend the noises they hear. Since the brain takes some time to acclimate to processing the electrical signals from the cochlear implant as meaningful sounds, consistent practice, and patience are essential.

Many people who utilize cochlear implants discover that they can lead happy lives and participate in activities that they previously thought were difficult or impossible. Appreciating music, engaging in group discussions, and even taking in peaceful noises like leaves rustling can become a regular part of their lives. Through the utilization of existing resources and opportunities, people with cochlear implants can fulfill their personal and professional objectives, leading to more fulfilling and socially engaged lives.